Hairdos

Hairdos

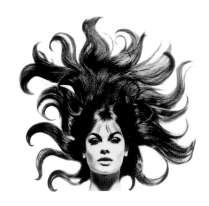

Stewart, Tabori & Chang

New York

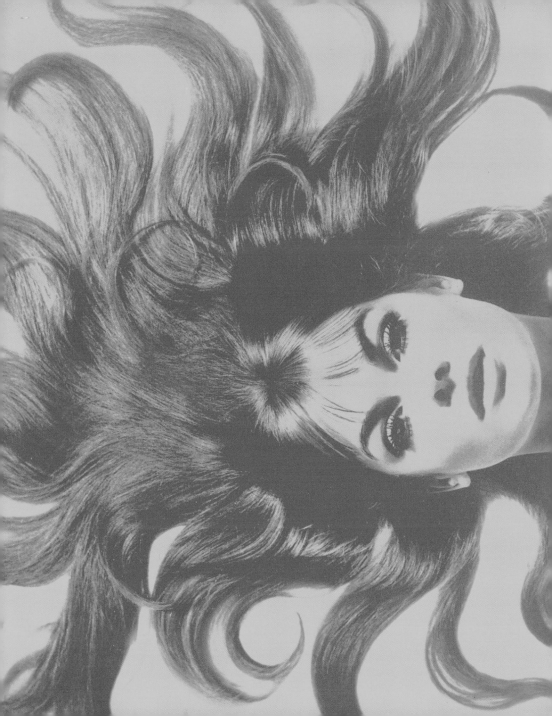

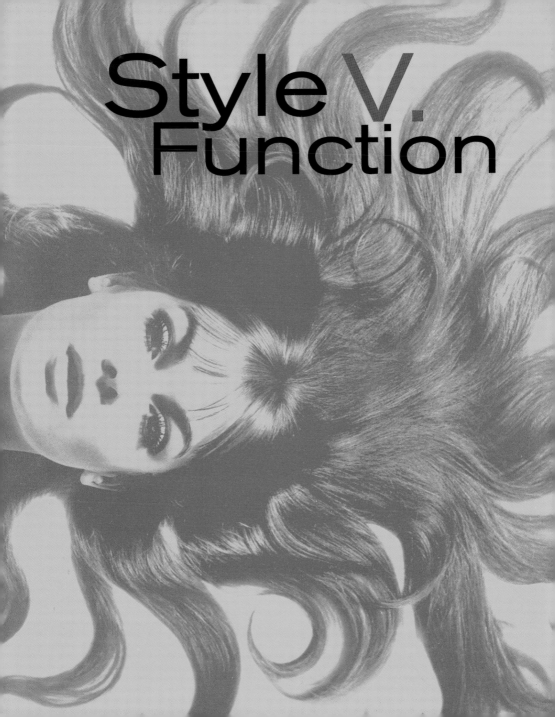

Style V. Function

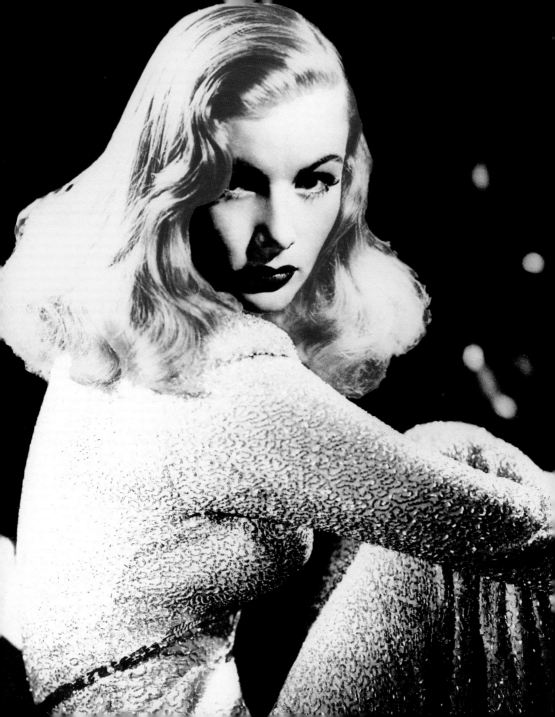

It was a blonde. A blonde to make a bishop kick a hole in a stained-glass window.

Raymond Chandler

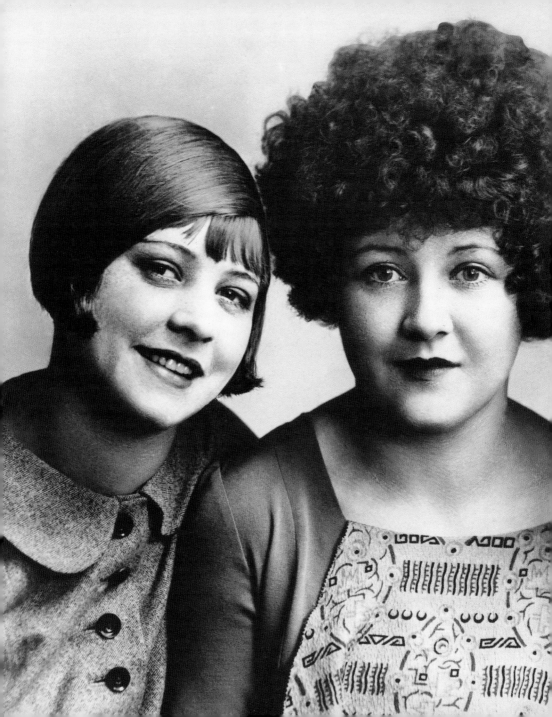

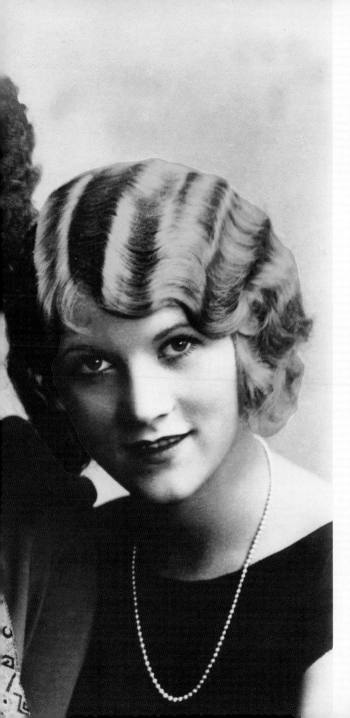

Violet will be
a good color
for hair at just
about the same
time that brunette
becomes a good
color for flowers.

FRAN LEBOWITZ

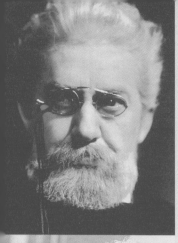

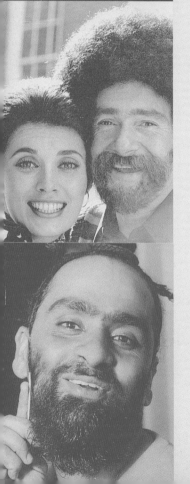

It always seemed
to me that
men wore their
beards, like
they wear
their neckties,
for show.

D.H. Lawrence

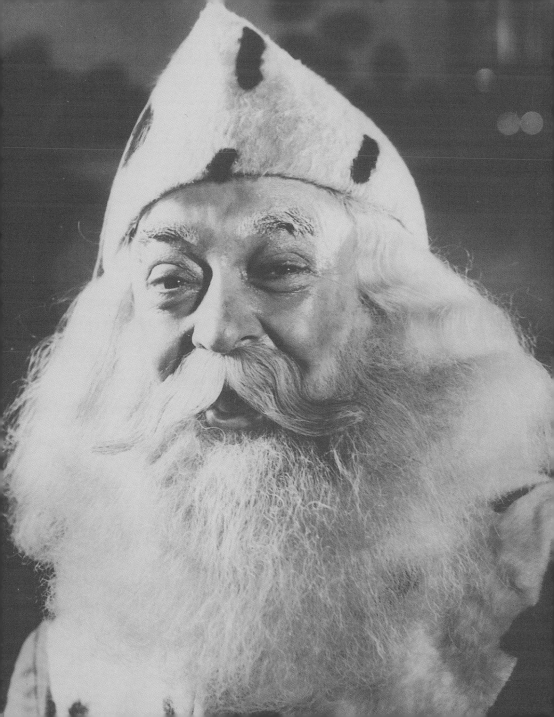

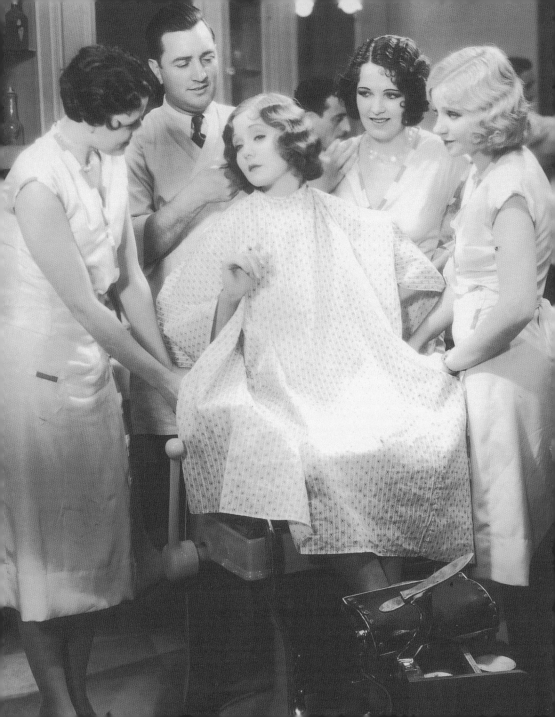

If truth is beauty,

how come no one

has their hair

done in the library?

LILY TOMLIN

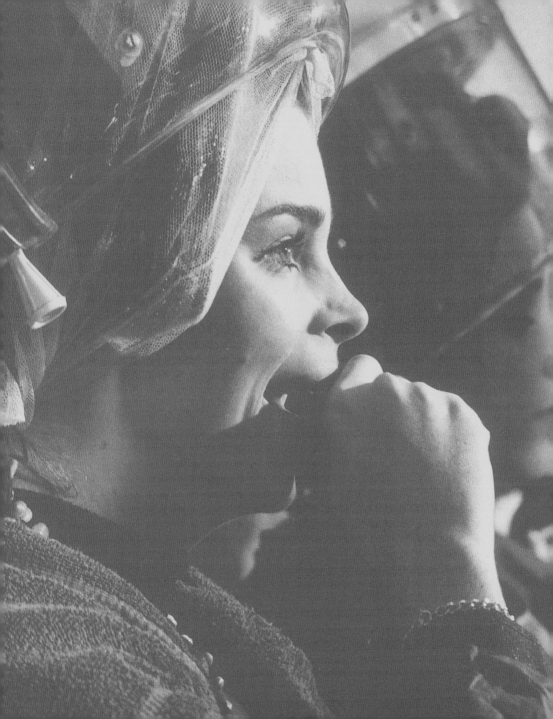

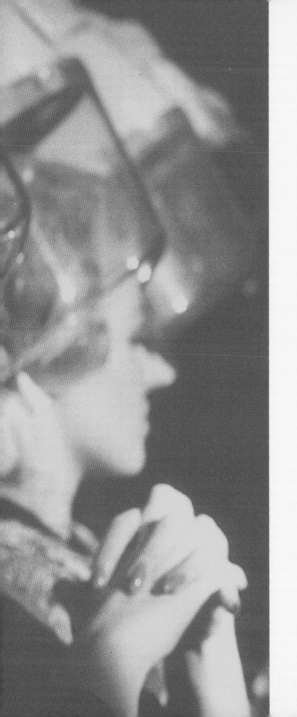

To Crystal, hair was the most important thing on earth. She would never get married because you couldn't wear curlers in bed.

Edna O'Brien

15

...Beware of
long arguments
and long beards...

GEORGE SANTAYANA

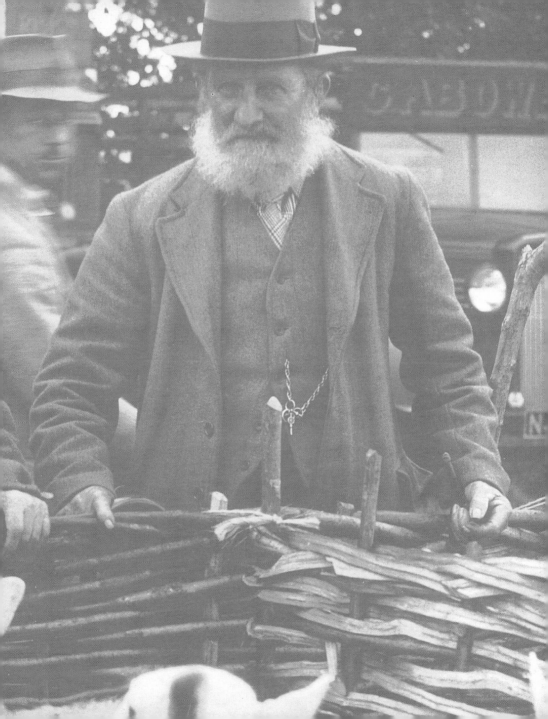

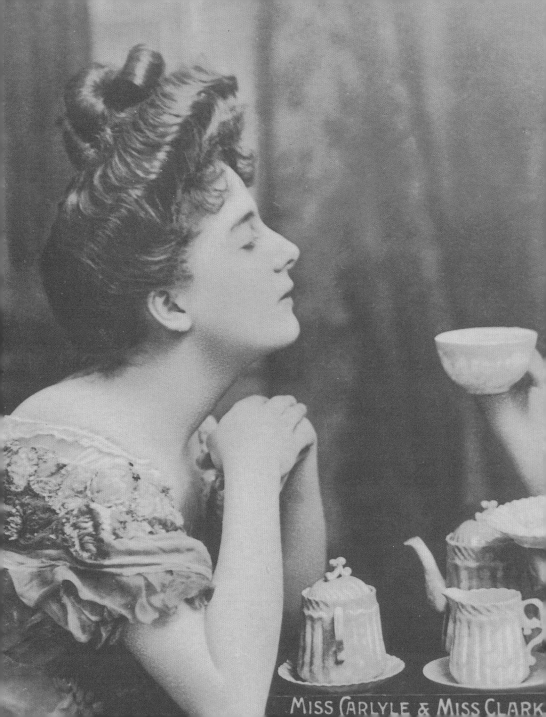

MISS CARLYLE & MISS CLARK

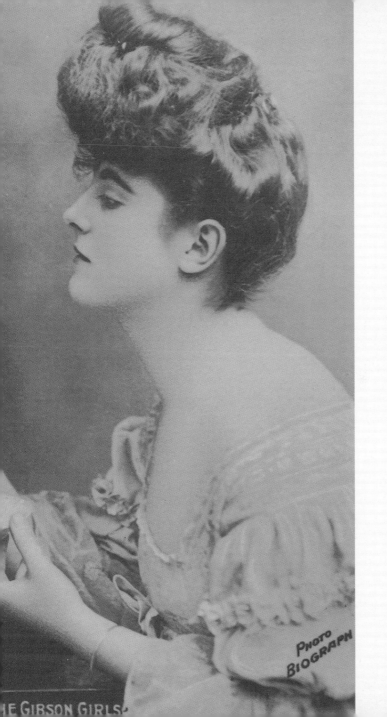

THE GIBSON GIRLS

PHOTO BIOGRAPH

HAIR RAISING

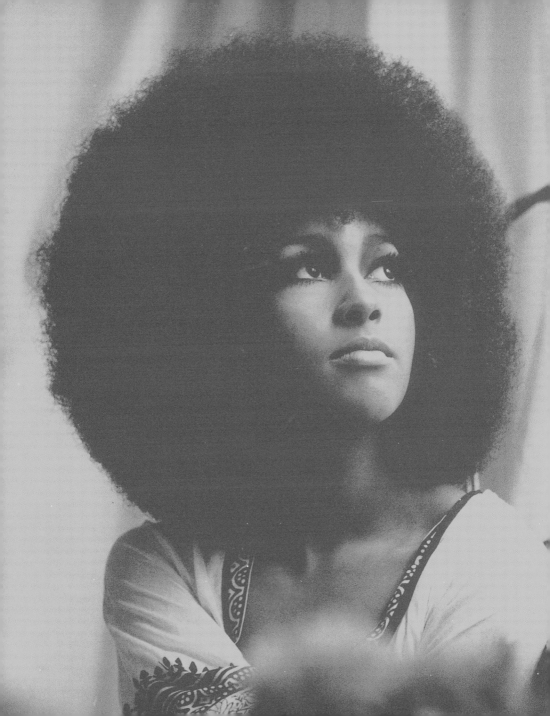

Long, *beautiful,* gleaming, steaming, flaxen, *waxen*... 'I adore hair!'

from the musical *HAIR*

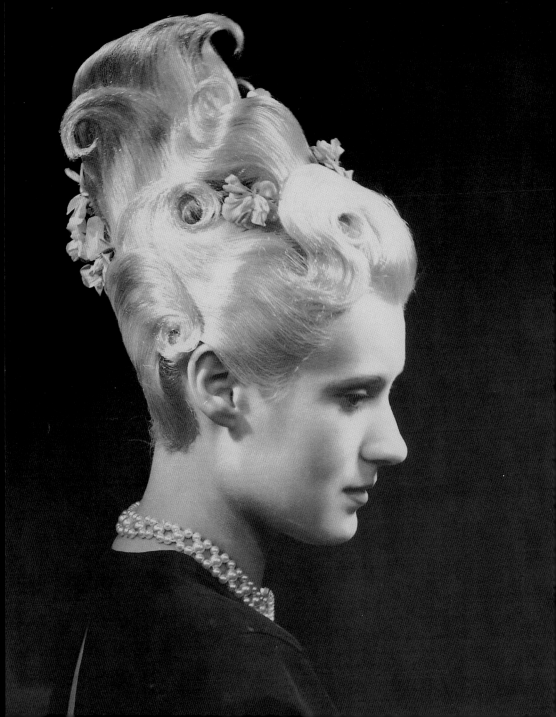

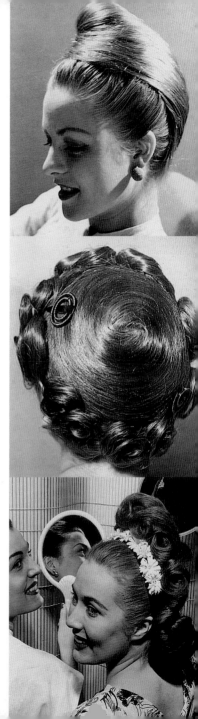

Only God, my dear,

Could love you for

yourself alone

And not your

yellow hair.

W.B. Yeats

There
is nothing
more contemptible
than a bald man who
pretends to have hair.

Martial, Epigrams

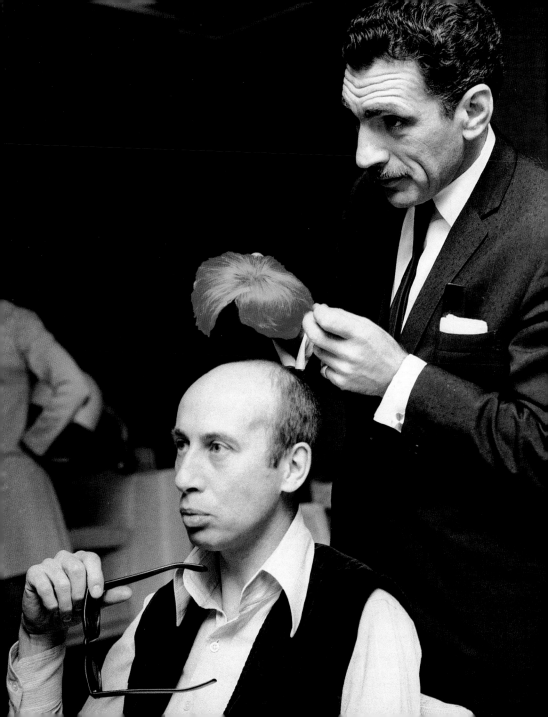

And, while she feels

the heavens lie

bare,

She only talks

about her hair.

FRANCIS THOMPSON,
THE WAY OF A MAID

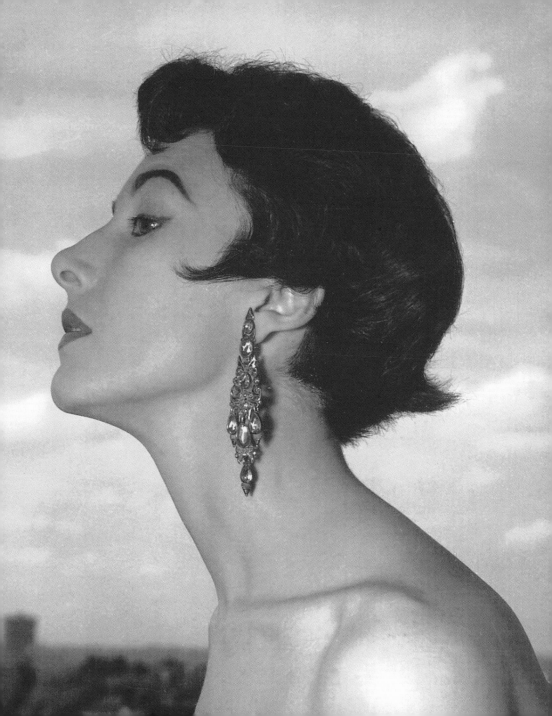

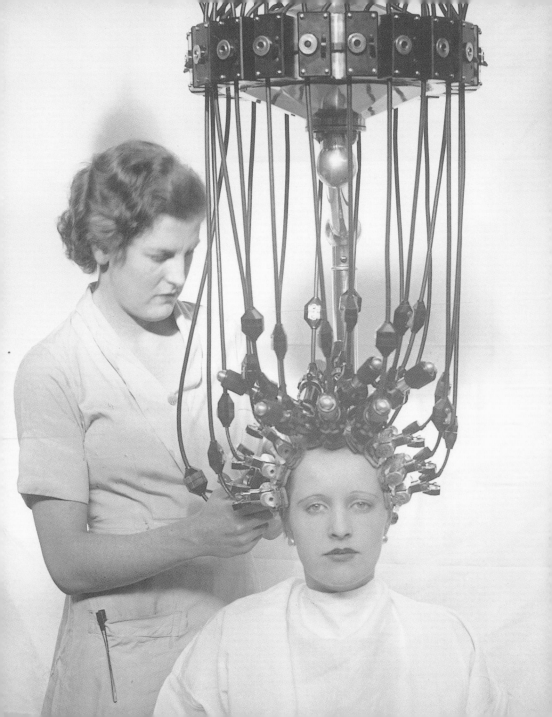

Everything is funny as long as it is happening to somebody else.

Will Rogers

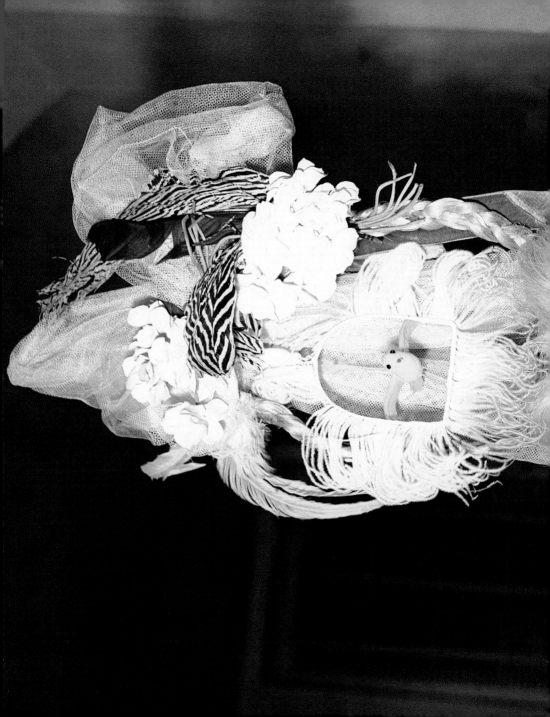

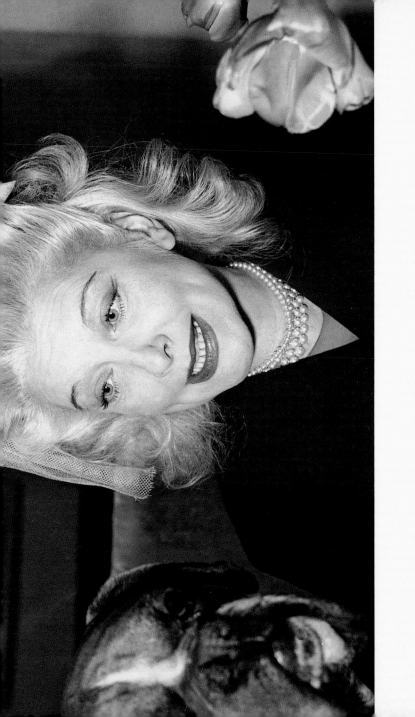

HAIRBRAINED

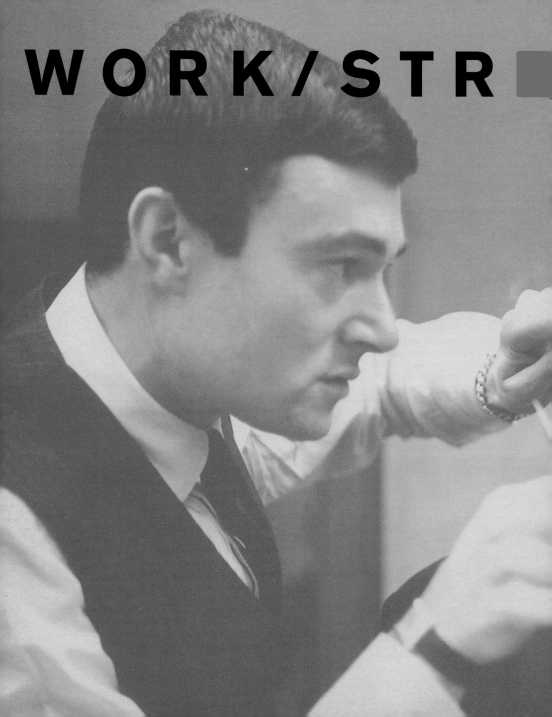

WORK/STR

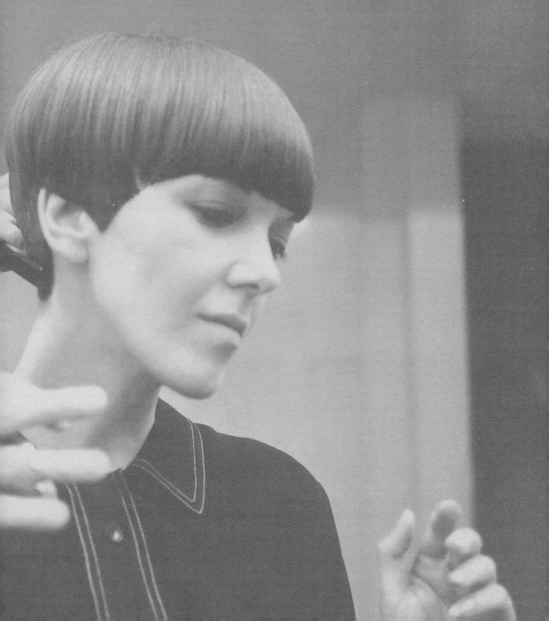

Beauty draws

us with a

single hair.

ALEXANDER POPE

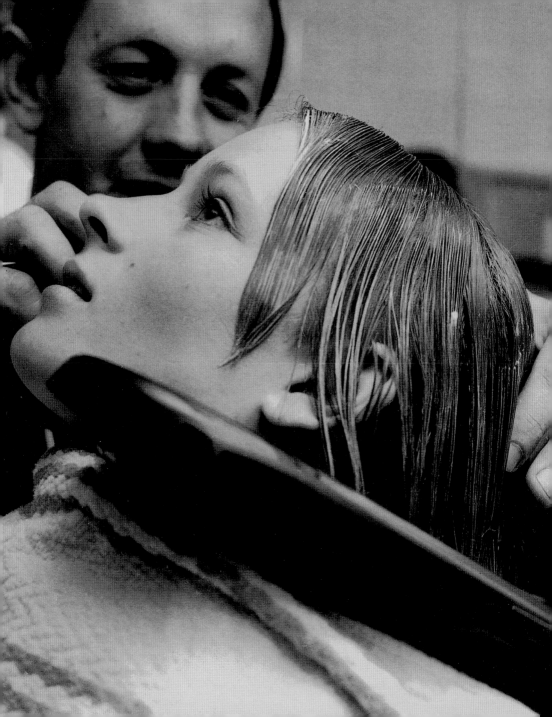

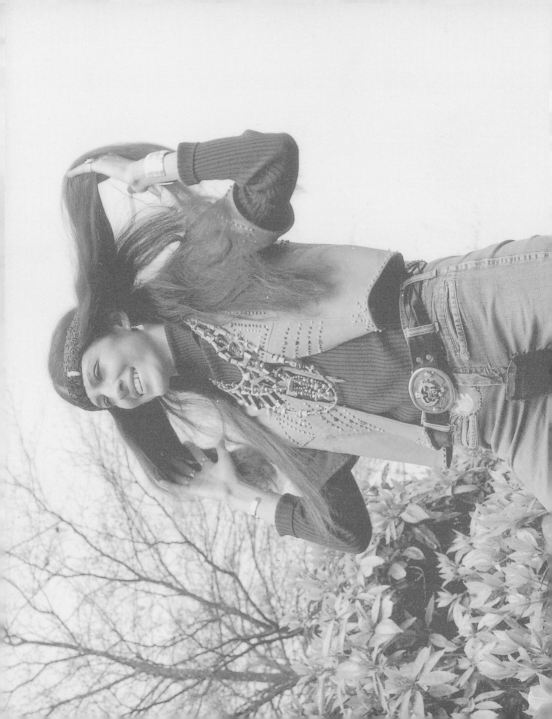

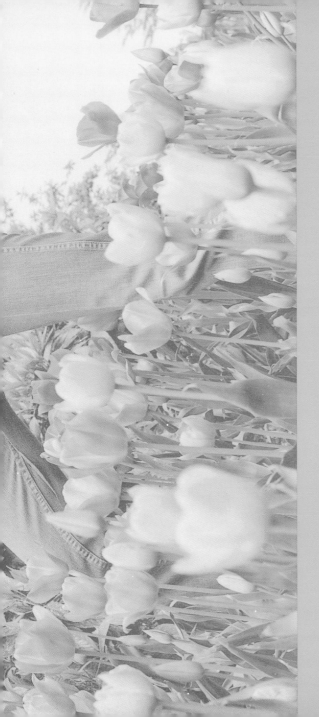

And forget not
that the earth
delights to feel
your bare feet
and the winds
long to play with
your hair.

Kahlil Gibran

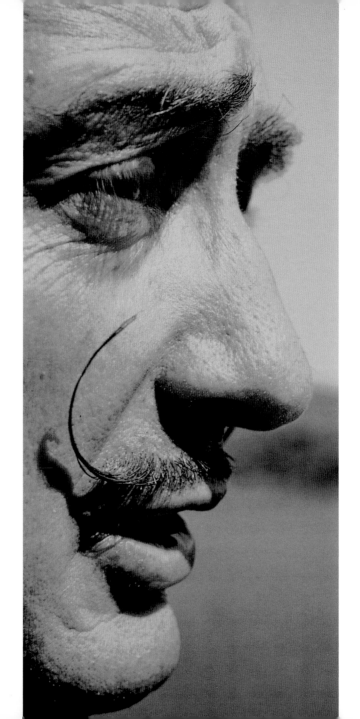

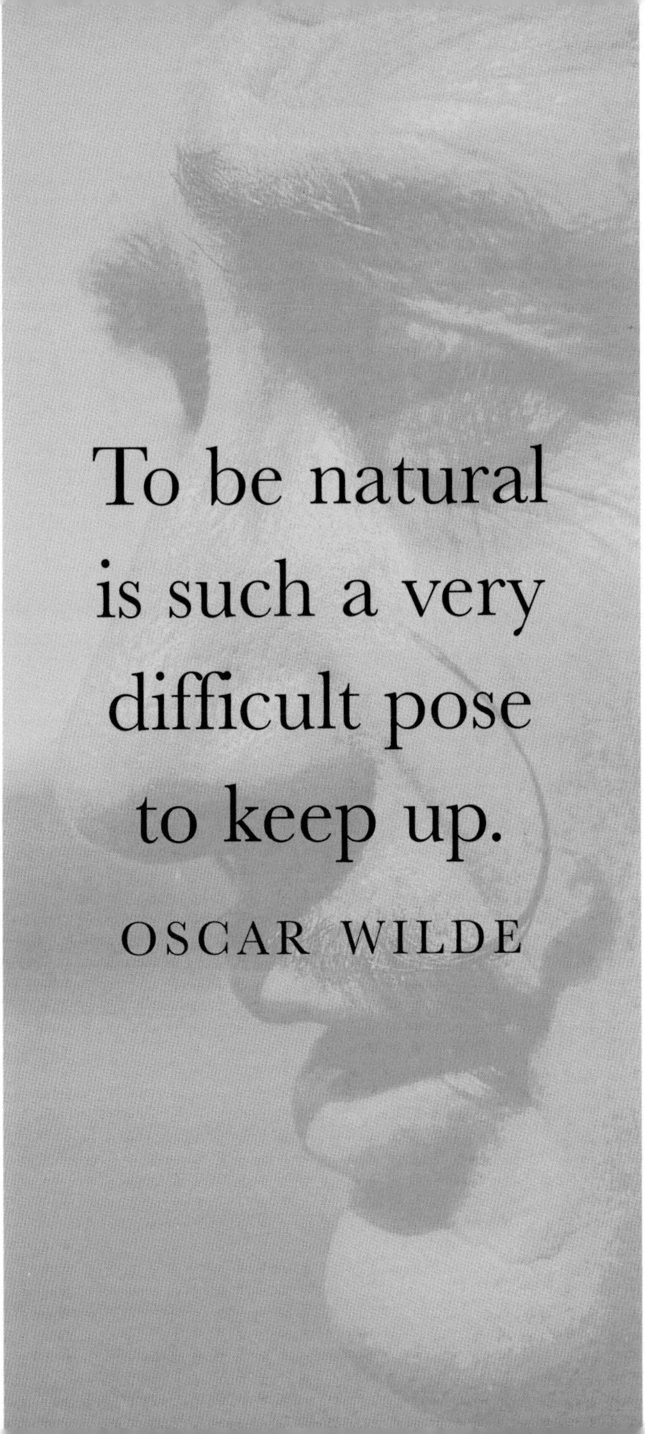

To be natural
is such a very
difficult pose
to keep up.

OSCAR WILDE

I see the
Beatles have
arrived from
England.
They were
forty pounds
overweight,
and that was
just their
hair.

Bob Hope

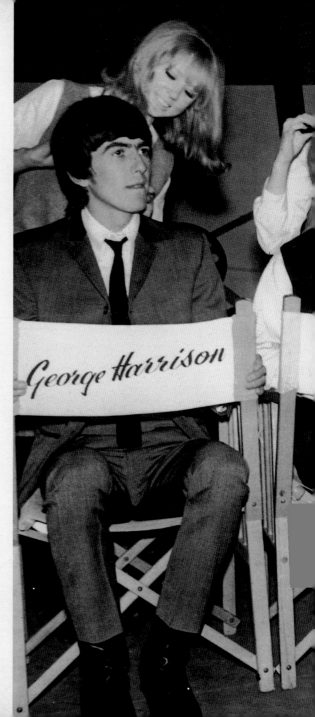

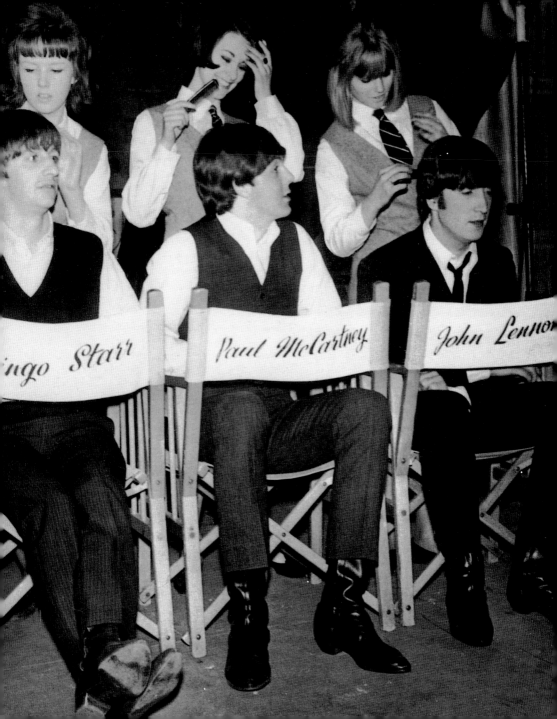

Between the cradle and the grave Lies a haircut and a shave.

Samuel Hoffenstein

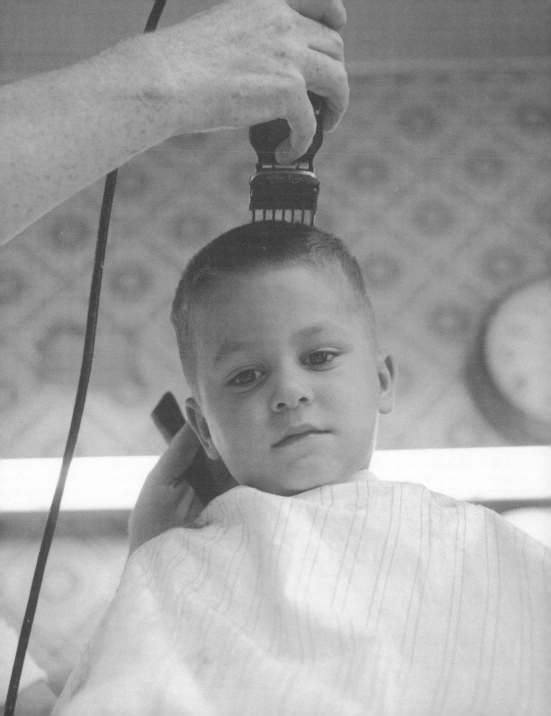

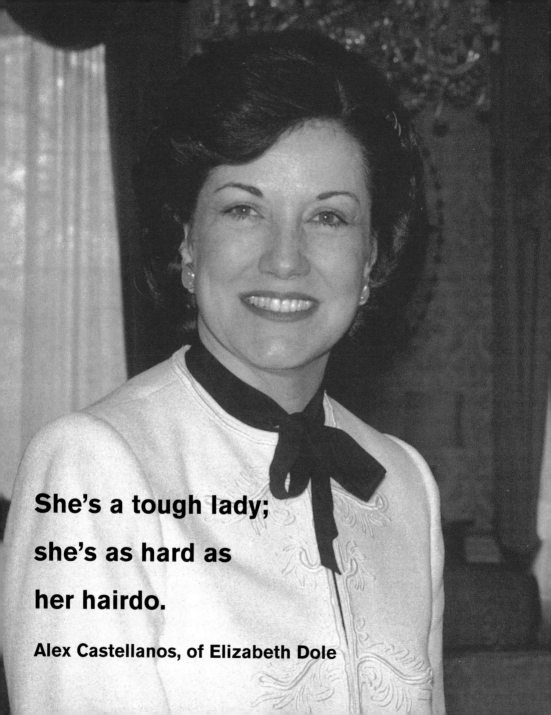

She's a tough lady; she's as hard as her hairdo.

Alex Castellanos, of Elizabeth Dole

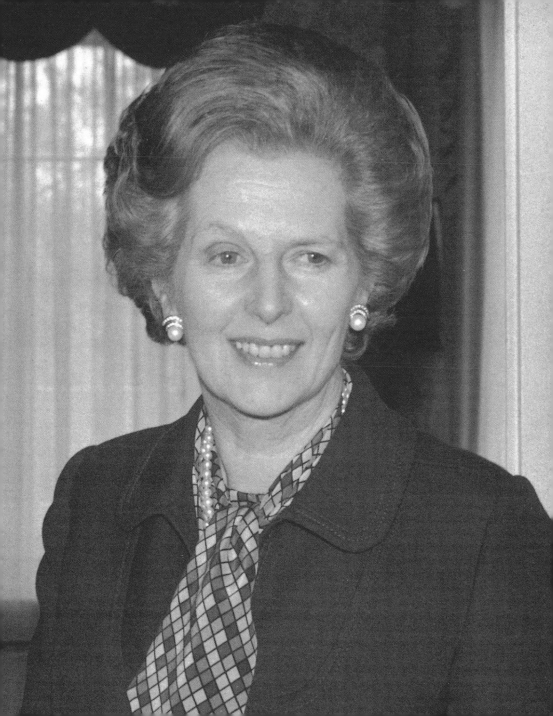

A fine head of hair adds
beauty to a good face,
and terror to an ugly one.

Lycurgus

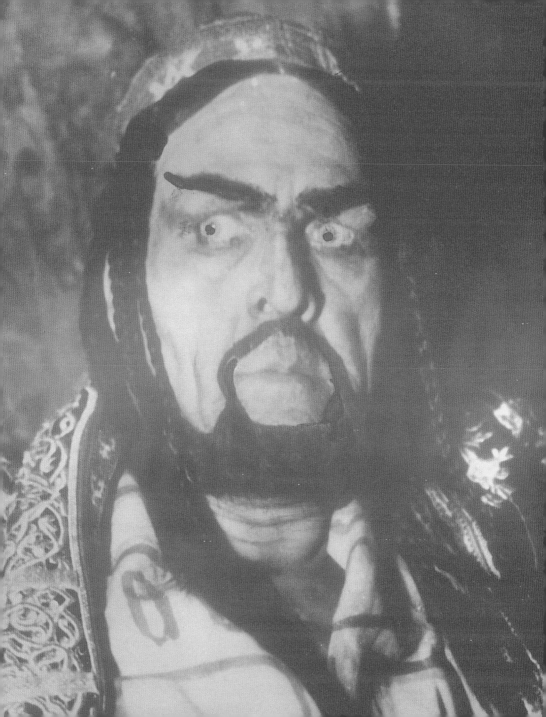

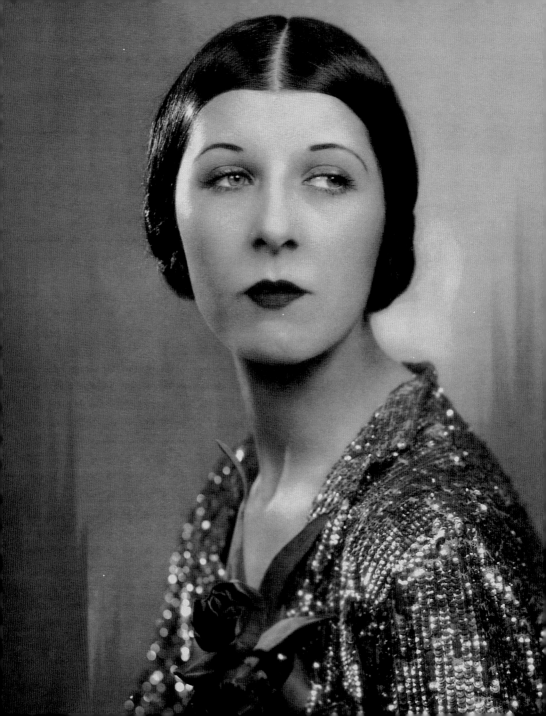

We flatten our hair on purpose to make it sleek and silky and to show the shape of our skulls, and it is our supreme object to have a head looking like a wet football on a neck as thin as a governess' hatpin.

Cecil Beaton

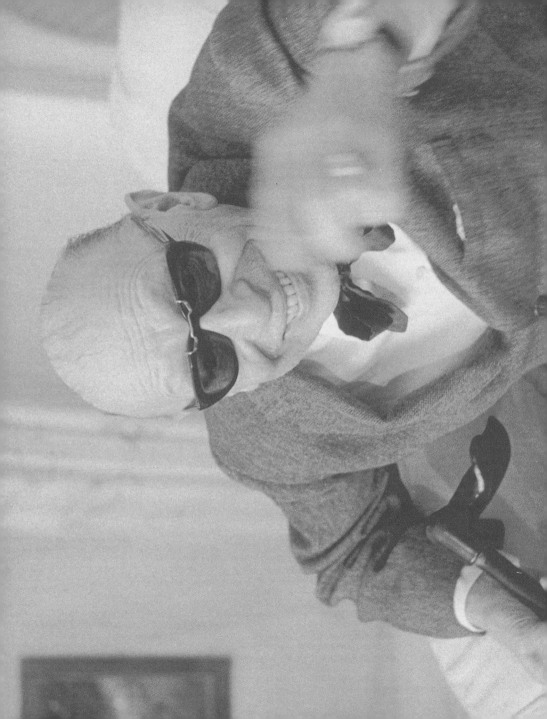

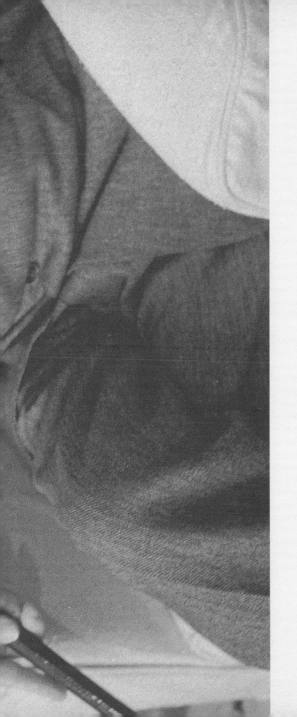

There is more felicity on the far side of baldness than young men can possibly imagine.

Logan Pearsall Smith

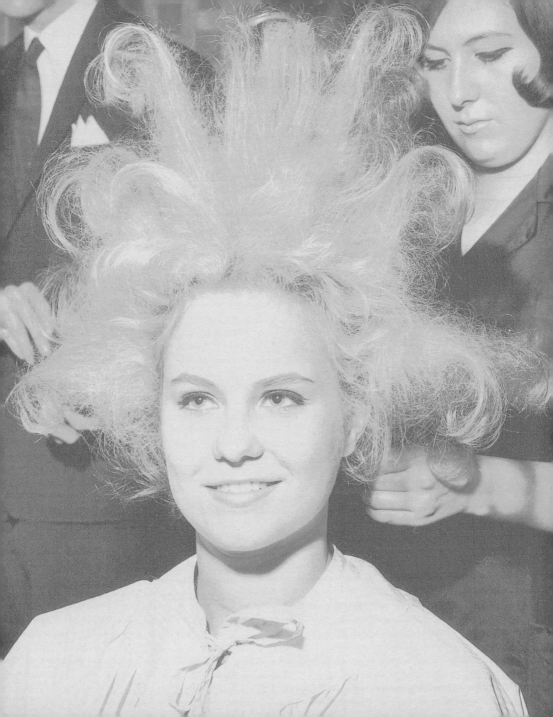

BAD
HAIR
DAY

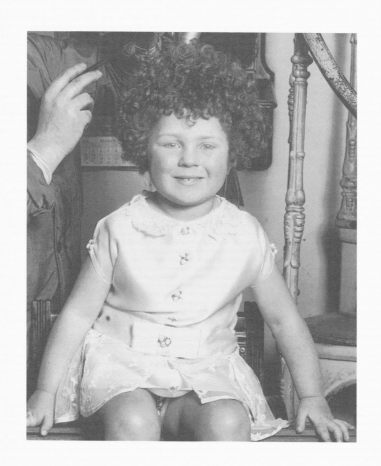

*T*here was a little girl,
Who had a little curl,
Right in the middle of her
forehead.

*A*nd when she was good,
She was very, very good,
And when she was bad,
she was horrid.

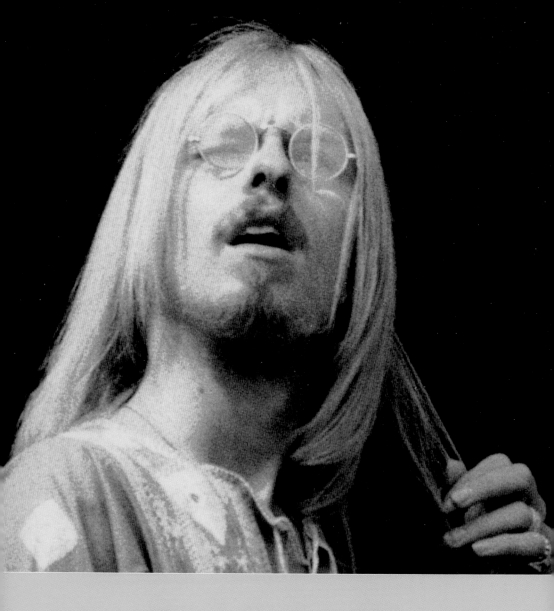

LOVE

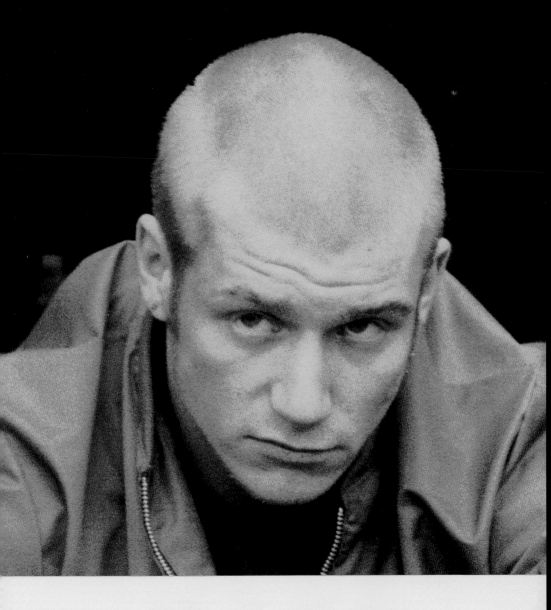

HATE

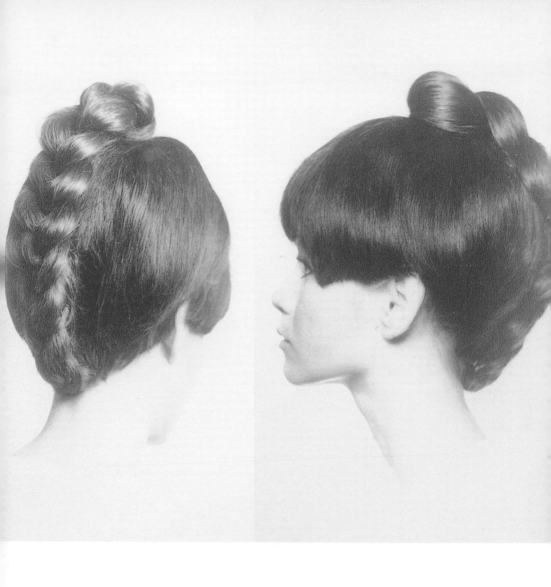

La Centurionne

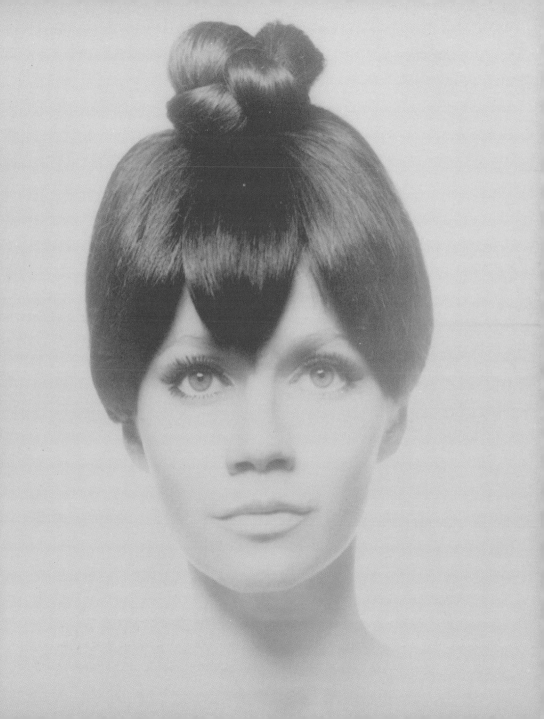

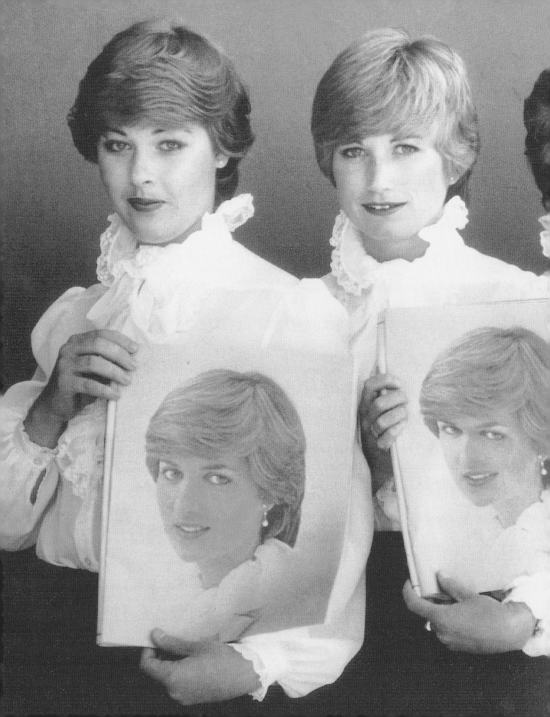

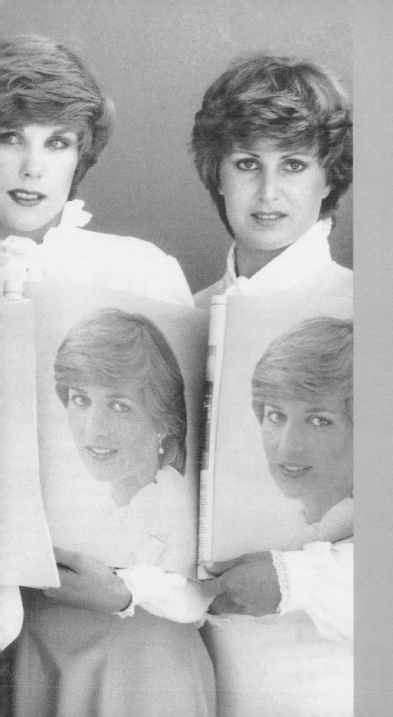

HAIR LINE

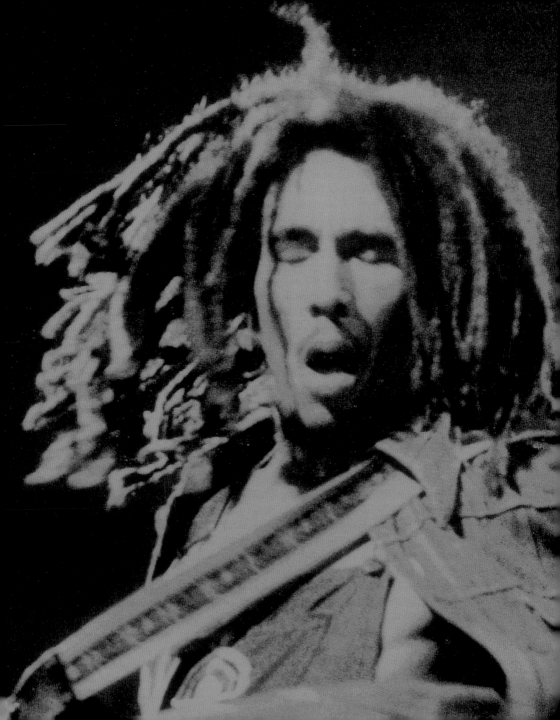

ICON

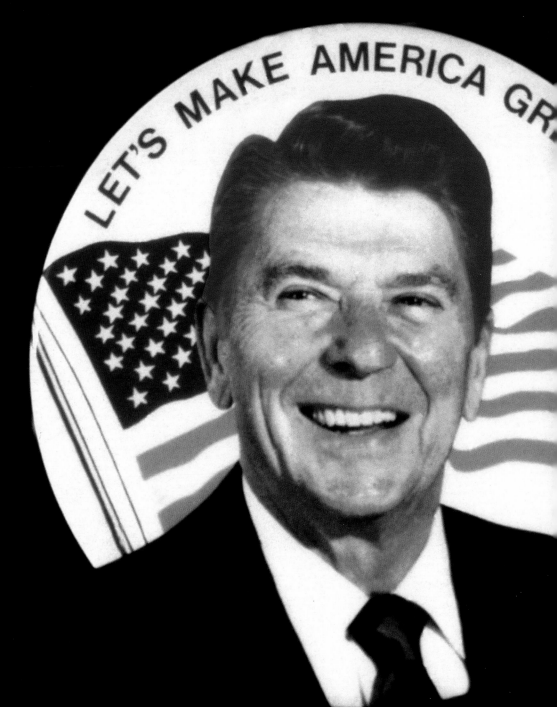

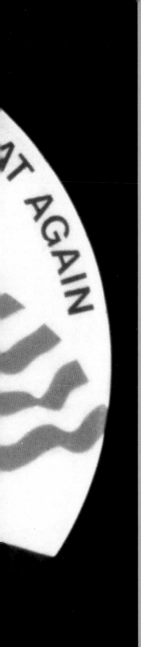

Ronald Reagan doesn't dye his hair, he's just prematurely orange.

Gerald Ford

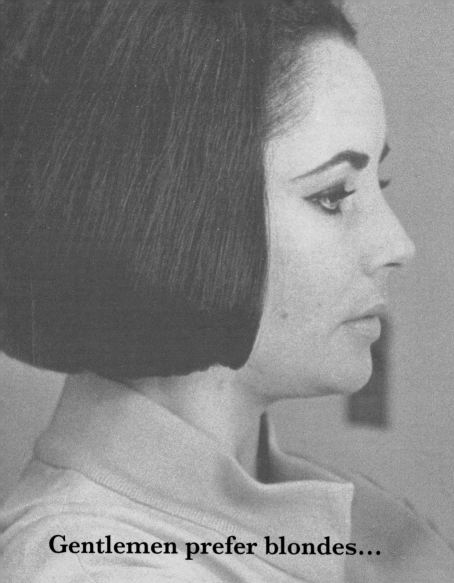

Gentlemen prefer blondes…

…but gentlemen marry brunettes

Anita Loos

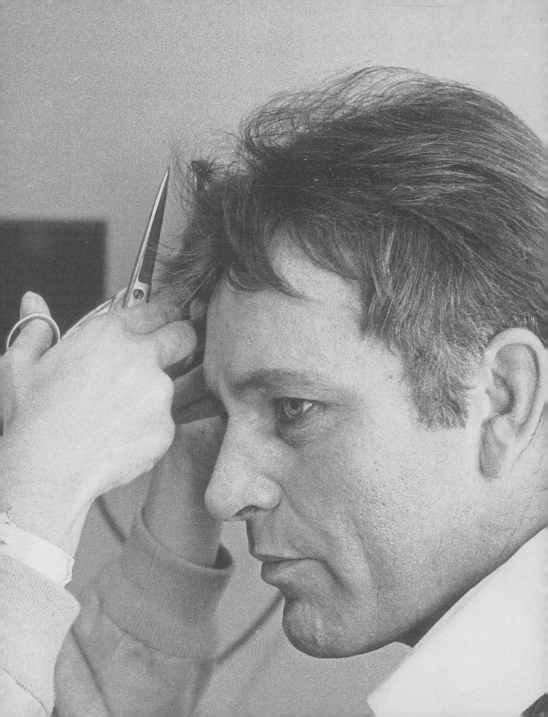

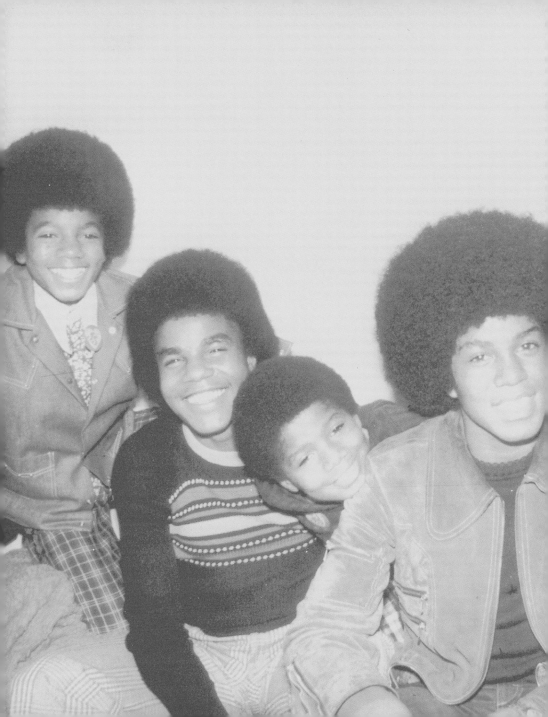

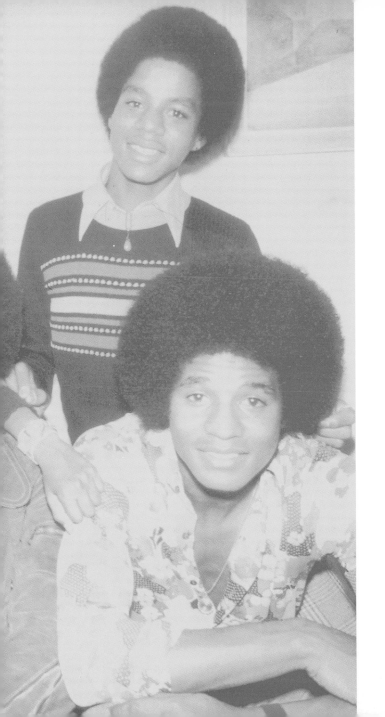

HAIR BAND

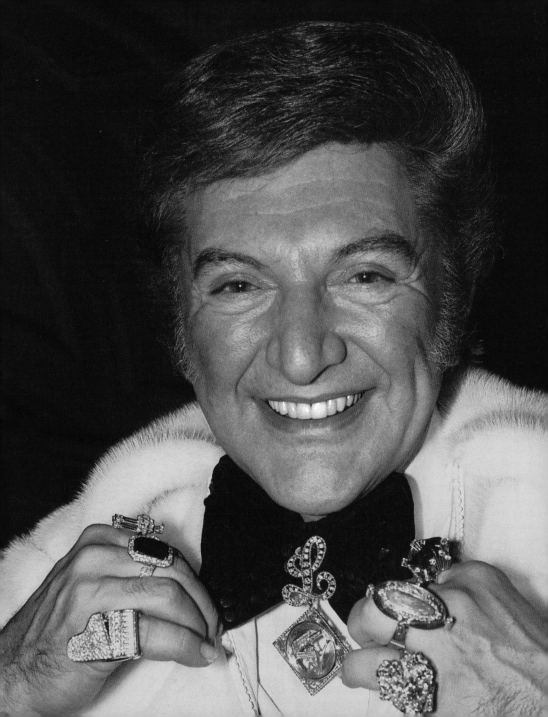

A celebrity is any well-known

T.V. or movie star who looks like

he spends more than two hours

working on his hair.

Steve Martin

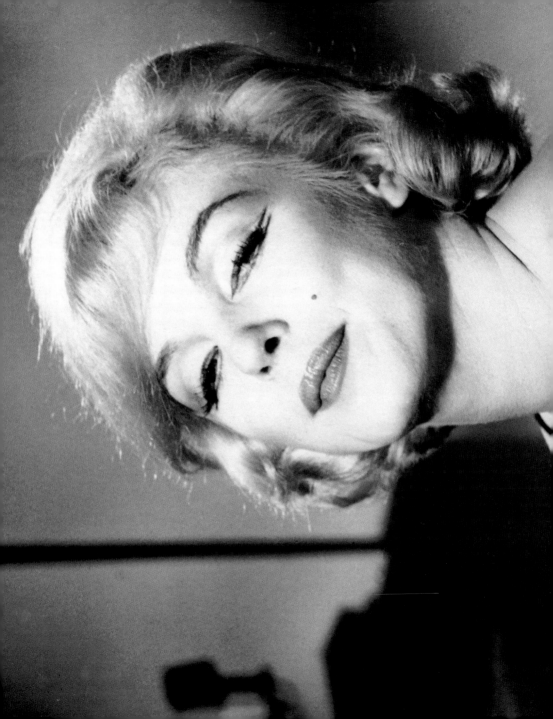

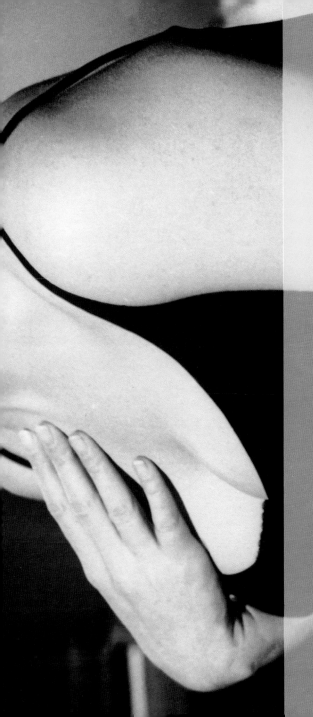

I may be a dumb blonde, but I'm not that blonde.

Patricia Neill

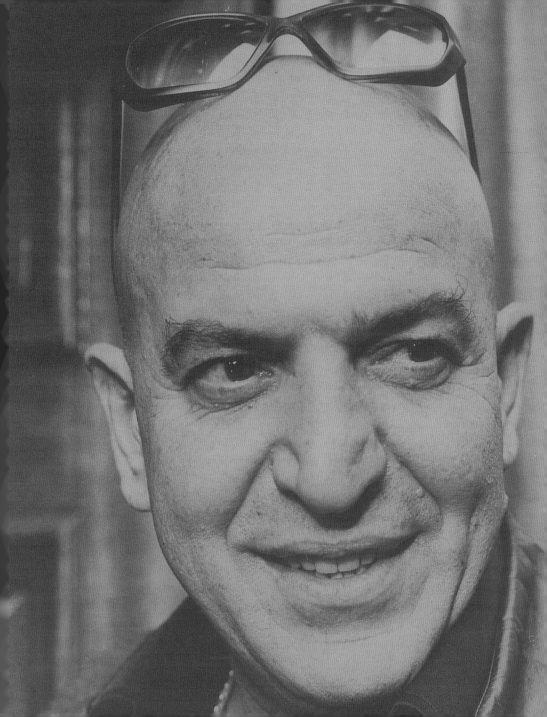

EGG-SHELL
BLONDE

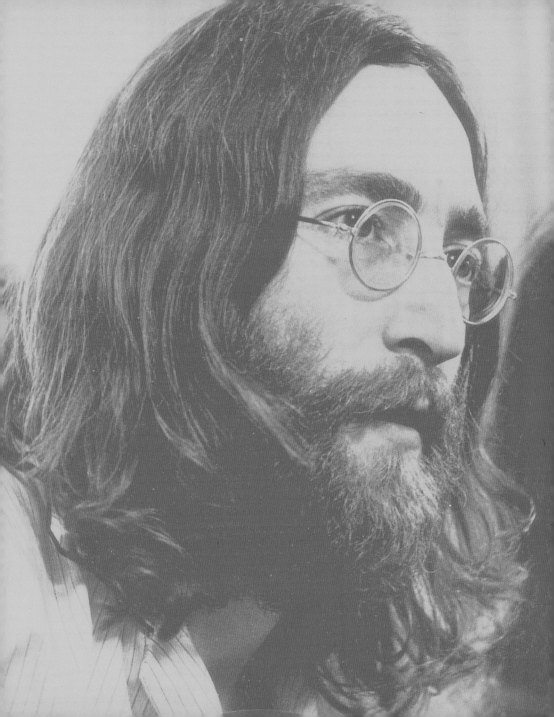

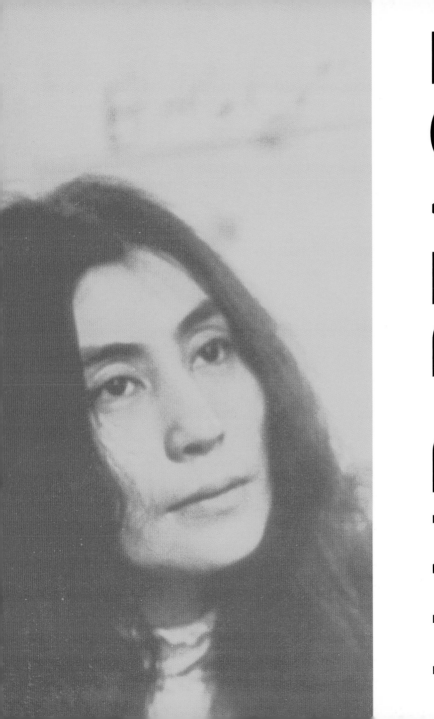

HAIR PEACE

PICTURE CREDITS

All images Hulton Getty Picture Collection.

cover, title page and page 4/5: Jean Shrimpton modelling the 'sun' hairstyle designed by Parisian hairstylist Carita, 1965.

page 6: Veronica Lake in a scene from the film 'I Wanted Wings', 1941.

page 8/9: Three women who feature in the play 'On With The Dance' at the London Pavilion, circa 1921.

page 10: From top to bottom, Danish actor Jean Hersholt, 1934, Vidal Sassoon, with his wife Beverly, 1972; Cricketer Bishen Bedi, 1977.

page 11: Father Christmas, 1960.

page 12: Nancy Carroll in a scene from the film 'Devil's Holiday', 1930.

page 14/15: Miss Canada, a 'Miss World' contestant, 1973.

page 16/17: Farmers at the Sussex sheep fair, 1936.

page 18/19: 'Gibson Girls', Miss Carlyle and Miss Clarke take tea, circa 1905.

page 20: Marsha Hunt, 1968.

page 22: Beryl Hardesty modelling a lacquered hairstyle, 1950.

page 23: From top to bottom, 'The Helmet' hairstyle, 1945; 'The Beehive' hairstyle, 1938; Hairstyle, 1949.

page 25: Man being fitted with a wig at Alexe's Queen Street salon, 1967.

page 26/27: 'The Spanish Cheekbone Curl' hairstyle, 1953.

page 28: Electric perming machine, 1935.

page 30/31: American actress Frances Day, 1949.

page 32/33: Mary Quant having her hair cut by Vidal Sassoon, 1964.

page 35: Heather Goldman having her hair styled by Robert Bowman, 1969.

page 36/37: American singer Rita Coolidge in Hyde Park, London, 1971.

page 38/39: Spanish surrealist artist Salvador Dali, 1951.

page 40/41: The Beatles, 1964.

page 43: Little boy having his hair trimmed with an electric shaver, 1955.

page 44/45: Elizabeth Dole (left) and Margaret Thatcher (right), 1984.

page 47: Russian bass singer Feodor Ivanovich Chaliapin as Prince Igor, circa 1890.

page 48: Nancy Beard, 1929.

page 50/51: Russian-born composer, conductor, pianist and writer Igor Fyodorovich Stravinsky, 1965.

page 52/53: Miss Finland, a 'Miss World' contestant, 1964.

page 54: Peggy Vaff modelling a 'bubble perm', 1930.

page 56: Hippy at the Isle of Wight pop festival, 1970.

page 57: Skinhead, Notting Hill, London, 1980.

page 58/59: 'La Centurionne', the French winter hairstyle of 1965.

page 60/61: Princess Diana lookalikes in New Zealand, 1984.

page 62/63: Bob Marley, 1975.

page 64/65: Ronald Reagan, 1980.

page 66/67: Elizabeth Taylor giving her future husband Richard Burton a haircut.

page 68/69: The Jackson Five, 1972.

page 70: Liberace, 1980.

page 72/73: Marilyn Monroe in a scene from the film 'Let's Make Love', 1960.

page 74: Telly Savalas, 1975.

page 76/77: John Lennon and Yoko Ono, 1969.

Published in 1999 by
Stewart, Tabori & Chang
A division of U.S. Media Holdings, Inc.
115 West 18th Street
New York, NY 10011

Distributed in Canada by
General Publishing Company Ltd.
30 Lesmill Road
Don Mills, Ontario, Canada M3B 2T6

Library of Congress Catalog Card Number: 98-88625

ISBN: 1-55670-934-X

Design: John Casey
Series Editor: Elizabeth Carr
Printed in Italy

10 9 8 7 6 5 4 3 2 1

The publishers are grateful to the following authors, agents and publishers for permission to reprint
the following copyright material:

Extract from the poem *For Anne Gregory* by W.B. Yeats reprinted by permission of A.P. Watt on
behalf of Michael B. Yeats.
Extract from *Hair*, music by Galt MacDermot. Words by James Rado and Gerome Ragni © 1966,
1967, 1968, 1970 James Rado, Gerome Ragni, Galt MacDermot, Nat Shapiro and EMI U
CATALOG INC, USA. Worldwide print rights controlled by Warner Bros Publications Inc/IMP Ltd.
All Rights Reserved.

Every effort has been made to contact copyright holders of material used.
In the case of any accidental infringement, concerned parties are
asked to contact the publishers.